The Remedy for Obesity

How to conquer food cravings,reduce weight and regain energy

By

Linda A. Ivey

Table of content

Introduction

Obesity is perhaps the single most dangerous factor to the general population's health in the United States, second only to smoking. The negative health impacts of obesity are widespread and extensive. They have a genuine and long-lasting influence not only on communities and countries but also, most crucially, on people, both now and in the generations to come.

Obesity is a leading cause of mortality among individuals under the age of 70 in the United States, second only to tobacco use in terms of the number of deaths it causes annually. The fatalities caused by obesity may soon surpass the deaths caused by tobacco use since tobacco use continues to fall, but obesity rates continue to grow. As with smoking, obesity either directly causes a large number of health conditions or is closely linked to a large number of health conditions. These conditions include coronary heart disease, stroke, diabetes, high blood pressure, unhealthy cholesterol, asthma, sleep apnea, gallstones, kidney stones, infertility, and as many as 11 types, including leukemia, breast, and colon cancer. The social and emotional implications of obesity are just as significant as the physical ones. These impacts include discrimination, lower income, reduced quality of life, and an increased likelihood of being susceptible to depression.

It encompasses many problems impacting society, including the national economy, productivity, and even national security. In 2005, obesity-related healthcare expenses in the United States might reach as high as $190 billion. This figure is more than twice that of prior predictions, and it is anticipated that these costs and obesity rates will continue to climb in the future decades. That includes money spent on medical treatment and prescription medicines directly connected to obesity. However, other expenses are related to obesity as well. These expenses include the cost of missed work days, increased insurance premiums for employers, and decreased salaries and incomes due to obesity-related diseases. Countries with lower obesity rates than the United States spend a lesser proportion of their healthcare budget on obesity-related issues. However, the burden is still a significant one. The impact of the current obesity epidemic in the United States on recruitment for the armed services is perhaps one of the most surprising consequences of the epidemic. According to the data, approximately 30 percent of young people in the United States are now too heavy to qualify for military service.

Chapter 1

factors associated with obesity

The situation known as obesity is characterized by an abnormally high amount of fat stored throughout the body. The matter of obesity is greater than just appearance. It is a condition that, when neglected, can lead to many infections and health problems, including those coronary infections, diabetes, high blood pressure, and even some forms of cancer.

There is a variety of factors that can contribute to someone having trouble losing weight. Obesity is generally caused by a combination of inherited, physiological, and environmental factors, as well as decisions regarding diet, level of physical activity, and exercise.

You might still gain weight even if you lead an active lifestyle and exercise regularly.

The good news is that even a moderate amount of weight loss can help improve or even prevent the health problems associated with obesity. Fixing your attitude, eating healthy meals, and exercising are all things that can help you lose weight.

Prescription Additional options for treating obesity include using weight-loss medications and surgical procedures.

To become less as one gets older. A slower metabolism is typically the result of having a smaller muscle mass. These changes also reduce the number of calories required, making it more difficult to maintain a healthy weight. If you don't calculatedly control what you eat and make an effort to become more physically active as you get older, you'll likely put on weight.

Other relevant aspects

- **Gaining weight:** during pregnancy is normal and should be expected. After giving birth, it can be challenging for some women to shed this additional weight. This weight gain may play a role in the progression of obesity in women.

- **Quitting smoking:** Giving up smoking is frequently associated with an increase in body mass. And for some people, it can cause weight gain severe enough to be classified as obesity. When someone is trying to deal with the withdrawal symptoms of smoking, they frequently turn to food for comfort.

  Nevertheless, if you want to improve your health in the long run, quitting smoking will be of greater benefit to you than continuing to smoke. After quitting smoking, your doctor should be able to assist you in maintaining a healthy weight.

- **Insufficiency in sleep:** Changes in hormones that cause an increase in appetite can be brought on by either not getting enough sleep or getting too much sleep. You may also find that you have an increased desire for foods that are high in calories and carbohydrates, both of which are factors that contribute to weight gain.

Numerous external factors can affect one's mood and well-being, and stress can be one of those factors. When under pressure, many people look for foods with a higher calorie content to comfort themselves. The meals you eat have an effect on the bacteria in your gut, which in turn may contribute to weight gain or make it more difficult to lose weight.

Even if you have any other dangerous factors, it does not necessarily mean that you will develop obesity at some point in your life. You can mitigate the effects of the majority of risk factors by making adjustments to your diet, your level of physical activity, exercise, and your behavior.

Complications

People who are obese have a high- risk of formulating some other potentially serious health issues, including the following:

Strokes and cardiovascular disease.

Being obese raises your risk of developing cardiovascular disease and stroke by increasing your likelihood of developing high blood pressure and abnormal cholesterol level. Both cases are dangerous factors.

Type 2 diabetes which insulin is utilized by the body to regulate blood sugar levels, can be disrupted by obesity. This increases the likelihood of developing insulin resistance as well as diabetes.

Certain cancers.

An increased body mass index is related with a high risk of developing cancer of the uterus, cervix, endometrium, ovary, breast, colon, rectum, esophagus, liver, gallbladder, pancreas, kidney, and prostate. Obesity also raises the risk of developing cancer of the esophagus.

Digestive problems:

The risk of developing conditions such as heartburn, gallbladder disease, and liver problems is increased by obesity.

Sleep apnea.

People who are obese have a high- risk of developing sleep apnea, a potentially life-threatening disorder in which the individual's breathing repeatedly stops and starts while they are asleep.

Osteoarthritis:

In addition to causing inflammation throughout the body, obesity places additional strain on the joints that are responsible for supporting the body's weight. These risk factors have the potential to result in complications like osteoarthritis.

Extremely severe symptoms of COVID-19.

If you become contaminated with the virus that caused coronavirus disease 2019, having a higher body mass index raises the likelihood that you will develop severe symptoms (COVID-19). Multitude who have severe cases of COVID-19 may require treatment in intensive care units or even mechanical assistance. These people may also have to seek assistance from other people.

Chapter 2

The calorie conundrum

It is accurate to say that the world we live in is preoccupied with calorie counting. Since the beginning of diet culture, the concept of calories, in conjunction with the "energy in, energy out" principle, has dominated the realm of wellness as a method for controlling body size and, purportedly, improving one's overall health.

It is logical and may even be appropriate to consider using calorie counting as a method to restore a healthy energy balance when it comes to recovering from hypothalamic amenorrhea (HA), relative energy deficiency in sport (RED-S), or a malnourishment disorder in the context of an energy deficit. These conditions all involve an energy deficit.

However, should you count calories when you are attempting to get your period back, and is there ever a time when it is genuinely suitable or helpful to do so?

This article intends to provide a review of the concept of calorie counting, including possible drawbacks and possible benefits to HA recovery. It is not my purpose to provide a definitive answer to the "calorie problem" for people who want to recover from missed periods; rather, I intend to provide you with the knowledge and insights that will enable you to decide what may work best for you. Simply put, what is a calorie?

A calorie is a unit of power that is equal to about 4.1868 joules of energy and can be loosely described as the quantity of heat needed to put forward the temperature of a quantity of water by one degree Celsius.

To put it plainly, the ability of our bodies to convert the energy contained in calorie-containing foods into other forms of energy that can be used by the body is the reason that we can continue living and the reason that our bodies can carry out all of the physiological and physical activities that are required of them, such as breathing, digesting food, thinking, and moving.

Typically, the quantity of energy that can be obtained from foods is measured in thousands of calories (kilocalories or kcal). On the other hand, given that "kilocalories" is such a cumbersome word to use, most people opt to use the phrase "calories" instead.

What are the drawbacks of keeping track of one's calorie intake?

Counting calories is a strategy that may be used to help you achieve your objectives and improve your health. There are various reasons why you might
want to give this strategy a close and careful look (including HA recovery).
The human body and its functions are not labs.
Because the concept that "a calorie is a calorie, is a calorie" is so ubiquitous, we frequently forget about the origins of these calories, the context in which they are found, and how they are utilized by the body.
You're likely familiar with the saying, "all calories are equal." However, although calories may be "equivalent" when they are outside of the body, this is not the case when they are inside the body. Because of important distinctions in food digestibility and food structure, the amount of energy that is included in specific foods (also known as their "calorie" content) may be different from the amount of energy that is theoretically computed. When comparing various foods with the same number of calories, it is important to keep in mind

that this does not necessarily mean that the effects of those foods on the body will be the same.

While it is true that the "system" of calories does, historically speaking, take into some consideration the processes involved in the digestion and absorption of calories from various foods and macronutrients, one cannot say the same thing about the metabolism of those foods. That is to say, various nutrients each contain their unique biochemical structures, which necessitate the use of distinct biochemical pathways and processes to extract the energy they contain.

One excellent illustration of this is provided by protein. Carbohydrates and proteins, gram for gram, have the same "value" in terms of their contribution to one's calorie intake. Both proteins and carbs have roughly the same caloric content per gram, though it should be noted that this figure is not exact.

However, once the calories in protein have been metabolized (the process of "releasing" energy that takes place after digestion and absorption), only 70% of those calories are available to be used as fuel for the body. However, the availability of the energy that is obtained from carbohydrates is only around 92%, whereas the availability of the energy that is obtained from fats is around 98%.

But let's look at still another illustration, shall we? Consider, for instance, the nuts of various trees. It's common knowledge that nuts have a high energy density in addition to a high-fat content (ranging between 40–75 g per 100 g). However, according to both experimental and observational research, including nuts as part of a balanced diet does not affect body weight (and, by extension, energy balance).

Mechanisms involving appetite control, dietary-induced thermogenesis (the amount of heat foods release in the process of extracting their

energy), and discrepancies in the amount of "food available energy" to the human body are some of the hypothesized reasons for this phenomenon. Other possible explanations include genetics and environmental factors.

As a result, you can see that the composition of a person's food has a significant influence in determining how precisely and successfully we can truly "count calories."

How we cook and eat our food makes a difference.

The subtleties of dietary composition and the energy (or caloric) availability of foods are further complicated by how humans choose, prepare, and eat various foods.

As was discussed before about the example of nuts, the presence of fiber, which is a category of complex carbohydrates that cannot be digested and is present in plants, makes it more difficult to break down food, hence lowering the amount of energy that is readily available from that food. Even natural variances in the state of food (such as whether we choose to eat green or yellow bananas, for example) can have some effect on the amount of energy that can be extracted from that food.

Cooking, blending, and juicing are just examples of the various preparation methods that can make a difference, and industrial processing processes, in particular, can make food more "accessible" to humans in terms of its energy content.

It also makes a difference in how we "combine" different foods. The glycemic load, which is a measurement of how much a particular food will elevate a person's blood glucose after they have eaten it, will change depending on whether we consume carbs on our own or in combination with proteins, fats, and fiber. This will, in turn, affect how we make use of and store that energy.

When you count calories without considering the context in which those calories were created in the food, the effects that different foods and their

combinations can have on our hormones, and even the chemistry in the brain that controls hunger and eating behaviors, you are missing important information.

Generic calorie prescriptions, such as 2000 kcal per day for women and 2500 kcal per day for men, are based on population averages that may not be relevant or hugely helpful in the context of individual health. Despite how wonderful it is to feel in control of our health with a daily calorie "quota," these generic calorie prescriptions are based on population averages. Simply put, each one of us has a wondrously singular personality (and vital force).

One of how this is manifested is in each of us unique bacteria of the gut (the microbial populations that live within our guts). In the past several years, new data has shown us that the microbial species in question have a significant influence on our capacity to extract energy from the food that we have eaten. The impact of the microbiota on the calorie

"currency" of food will vary from person to person, even though the extent to which we can (and should) influence this internal ecosystem to promote health is not yet fully known. This is although we are aware of the need to do so.

A daily calorie prescription will not take into account the daily changes in energy need that each body would experience. This is another crucial issue that must be taken into account. Multiple causes, such as non-exercise-induced activity thermogenesis (NEAT), emotional stress, temperature adaptations, physiological changes (such as having a monthly cycle), and recovery from injury or illness, are all contributors to these changes.

Last but not least, a person who has been surviving on a very low daily calorie intake before beginning the process of recovering from a condition of malnutrition may require a great deal more energy than is often taken into account. This "extra" energy will be required to help restore the healthy function of a variety of physiological processes, as well as makeup for the hypermetabolism that may occur as a result of this process (a state in which metabolism will speed up to capture the increase in energy supplied). Both of these goals must be accomplished before the "extra" energy can be considered useful.

When evaluating the efficacy of calorie tracking, it is essential to remember the significance of pleasure and the degree to which one feels satisfied by the food one eats.

My experience dealing with customers has shown me that we frequently seek to reinstate a more natural, playful, and inquisitive relationship with food. In other words, we want to put the joy back on the menu. In my opinion, one of the finest ways to ruin the fun is to make the process of eating into some kind of complicated math problem.

Simply put, calories are not the same thing as pleasure.

In addition, if an individual has reached a state of malnourishment, relative energy shortage, or HA by placing a strong focus on calorie "management" (whether self-imposed or otherwise), then we need to seriously evaluate together if counting calories is the way to recovery.

I am aware that in the beginning, having a "ballpark" number to target or a calorie goal might be useful for many different types of women. However, it is crucial to note that counting calories eliminate the instinctive and intuitive capacity to construct and balance a meal that is both satiating and nourishing.

When it comes to HA recovery, can tracking calories serve any useful purpose?

Regardless of whether or not I was able to address your question in the previous paragraph, the responsibility ultimately lies with you.

If you're in a situation in which you're feeling lost, it may be beneficial to strive for a minimal number; nevertheless, once you've hit that minimum, it's strongly recommended that you stop counting the remainder of the items.

I would advise you to cease tracking calories as soon as you feel comfortable planning meals and selecting foods to support your daily consumption following that quotient.

Calories (as soon as possible) to facilitate a speedier return to a place of intuitive eating concerning food. Be patient.

A continued focus on the "numbers," such as calories consumed or burned, weight, or steps taken, risks serving the underlying beliefs and behaviors that have led to HA or relative energy deficiency rather than the true values or goals of recovery.

*It is important to note that there is no single quotient; therefore, I suggest consulting with a registered nutrition professional who specializes in this area to assist in determining a starting point that is both safe and attainable. If you are working by yourself, you should aim to consume at least 2,000 kcal per day (please then stop counting). When it comes to patients who have HA, a common piece of advice that can be found in the scientific literature is to aim (initially) for a 5% increase in body weight, which can lead to period recovery and improve bone mineral density.

Chapter 3

The mechanisms of obesity involving hormones

Hormones are essential substances that play an important role in the body by acting as chemical messengers.

They play a role in almost every physiological process, including the regulation of metabolism, hunger, and satiety. Some hormones play a significant role in weight regulation because of their connection to appetite and other functions.

This article will discuss nine hormones that may influence your weight and provide suggestions for maintaining healthy levels of those hormones.

1. Insulin: Your pancreas is responsible for producing insulin, which is the primary storage hormone in your body. Insulin encourages the storage of glucose in otherwise healthy individuals.

A type of sugar that can be stored in the body's skeletal muscle, liver, and adipose tissue for later use.

Insulin is secreted by your body in smaller amounts periodically throughout the day and in greater quantities after meals. This hormone then transfers glucose from the food you eat into your cells, then it can either be used for power or reserved, depending on the requirements of your body at the moment.

Insulin resistance is a condition that affects a significant portion of the population and occurs when your cells stop responding to insulin. Because insulin is unable to transport glucose into the cells, while you have this condition, you will have high blood sugar.

After that, your pancreas will produce even more insulin to improve your body's ability to absorb glucose.

Insulin resistance has been correlated to obesity, which can play a role in other situations, such as type 2 diabetes and heart disease. Obesity has been linked to insulin resistance.

Insulin sensitivity can be presumed to the contrary to insulin resistance. Insulin resistance can be caused by diabetes. It indicates that your cells are receptive to the hormone insulin. As an outcome, it is a wise decision to concentrate on lifestyle habits that help enhance insulin sensitivity, such as the ones that are listed below.

Suggestions to increase insulin responsiveness

- **Exercise regularly.** Whether performed at a high or moderate intensity, exercise has been shown to improve insulin sensitivity while simultaneously reducing insulin resistance. This is supported by research.
- **Change your sleeping patterns for the better**: There is a correlation between not getting enough sleep or not getting quality sleep and obesity and insulin resistance.

According to some research, taking omega-3 supplements may help people with metabolic conditions such as diabetes become more sensitive to the effects of insulin. If you don't like taking supplements, you could try increasing the amount of fish, nuts, seeds, and plant oils that you eat instead.

- **Change your diet:** There is some evidence that the Mediterranean diet, which features a high intake of vegetables along with healthy fats obtained from nuts and extra-virgin olive oil, can help reduce insulin resistance. It's possible that reducing your consumption of saturated and trans fats will also be beneficial.

- **Keep your weight at a healthy level:** Insulin sensitivity may be improved in people who are overweight by engaging in healthy weight loss and by managing their weight.

- **Focus on foods that are low in glycemic index:** Instead of trying to cut carbohydrates out of your diet entirely, focus on making the majority of them low glycemic and high in fiber. Whole grains, fruits, vegetables, and legumes are some examples of nutritious foods.

2. Leptin

The hypothalamus, which is the part of your brain that controls appetite, receives the signal that you are full from the hormone leptin, which tells it that you are no longer hungry. On the other

hand, those who are obese are more likely to have leptin resistance. This means that the signal to your brain

to stop eating does not get through, which will eventually lead to you overeating.

As a result, your body may produce even more leptin until it reaches a level where it is considered high.

It is not clear what the direct cause of leptin resistance is; however, it could be due to inflammation, gene mutations, or excessive leptin production, which is something that can happen when someone is obese.

Suggestions to Help Raise Your Leptin Levels

Although there is currently no known treatment for leptin resistance, making a few changes to your lifestyle could help lower leptin levels:

It is important to keep a healthy weight because leptin resistance is associated with obesity, and maintaining a healthy weight can help prevent obesity. In addition, research has shown that a

reduction in body fat may assist in lowering levels of the hormone leptin.

- **Enhance the quality of your sleep:** Leptin levels may be related to the quality of sleep experienced by people who are obese. Even though this correlation might not hold for people who aren't overweight, there are still plenty of other good reasons to improve your sleeping habits.

- **Exercise regularly:** According to research, engaging in regular and consistent exercise can lead to a reduction in levels of the hormone leptin.

3. Ghrelin

Ghrelin can be thought of as the antithesis of the hormone leptin. It is the hunger hormone that conveys to your hypothalamus the information that your stomach is bare and requires nourishment to function properly. Its primary purpose is to stimulate hunger and appetite.

In a normal person, the levels of the hormone ghrelin are at their highest just before eating and at their lowest right after eating.

Research has shown that people who are overweight have lower levels of the hormone ghrelin, but they are more sensitive to the effects of the hormone. Because of this sensitivity, one might end up eating excessively.

Advice for controlling your body's ghrelin levels

One of the reasons why losing weight can be challenging is because reducing calorie intake frequently results in increased ghrelin levels, which leaves you feeling hungry. The metabolism also tends to slow down, and the levels of the hormone leptin tend to fall.

As a result, the following are some suggestions for reducing ghrelin, which can also help reduce appetite:

It's important to keep your weight in check because being overweight can make you more exposed to the hormone ghrelin, which can ultimately make you hungrier.

- **Make an effort to get some restful sleep.** Inadequate sleep has been linked to increases in the hunger hormone ghrelin, as well as overeating and subsequent weight gain.
- **Eat regularly:** Because levels of ghrelin are at their highest just before a meal, it is important to pay attention to cues from your body and eat when you feel hungry.

4. Cortisol

Your adrenal glands are accountable for producing cortisol, which is commonly referred to as the stress hormone.

This hormone is responsible for the increased heart rate and levels of energy that are experienced in

times of high stress. The "fight or flight" response is another name for the simultaneous release of the hormone adrenaline and the stress hormone cortisol.

While it is essential for your body to release cortisol in dangerous situations, chronically high levels have been linked to a variety of adverse health effects, such as diabetes, heart disease, low energy levels, high blood pressure, sleep disturbances, and increased body mass.

It's possible that having high cortisol levels is caused in part by certain aspects of one's lifestyle, such as not getting enough sleep, being under constant stress, and eating a lot of foods with a high glycemic index.

In addition, not only does obesity cause cortisol levels to rise, but high cortisol levels may also cause individuals to gain weight, thereby creating a vicious cycle.

Suggestions for bringing down your cortisol levels

The following are some changes in lifestyle that may assist in cortisol level management:

- **Optimize sleep:** Chronic sleep problems such as insomnia, sleep apnea, and irregular sleep habits (such as those of shift workers) have been linked to elevated levels of the stress hormone cortisol. Make it a priority to establish a consistent time for going to bed and getting up.

- **Exercise regularly**: Intense exercise causes a transient rise in cortisol levels, whereas moderate-to-vigorous exercise on a more consistent basis helps reduce cortisol levels by enhancing overall health and mitigating the negative effects of stress.

- **Mindfulness training should be done:** There is preliminary evidence that frequent practice of mindfulness can reduce cortisol levels, but

  this area of study has to be expanded. Consider incorporating meditation into your typical regimen.
- **Keep your weight in the healthy middle range**: Maintaining a healthy, normal weight may help keep cortisol levels under control. Obesity has been linked to increased cortisol levels, and high cortisol levels have been linked to weight growth.
- **Consume food from each food group:** According to the findings of certain studies, diets that are heavy in added sugars, refined carbohydrates, and saturated fat may result in increased levels of the stress hormone cortisol. In addition, following a diet similar to that of the Mediterranean may assist in reducing cortisol levels.

5. Estrogen: Estrogen is a kind of sex hormone that controls not just the reproductive system of females but also the immunological system, the skeletal system, and the cardiovascular system.

The levels of this hormone fluctuate not just throughout the menstrual cycle but also the many periods of life, such as pregnancy, lactation, and menopause.

People who are obese tend to have high amounts of estrogen, which is connected with an increased risk of some cancers and other chronic diseases. Obese people also tend to have higher levels of other hormones called androgens.

On the other hand, low levels, which are often associated with aging, perimenopause, and menopause, are known to impact body weight and body fat, hence increasing the likelihood that you may suffer from chronic diseases.

Central obesity, which refers to an accumulation of weight around the trunk of the body, is a condition that frequently affects people whose estrogen levels are low. This can result in a variety of other health issues, including hyperglycemia, hypertension, and coronary heart disease.

Modifications to your lifestyle, most notably the maintenance of healthy body weight, can help you reduce your chance of developing many of these diseases and disorders.

Advice on how to keep your estrogen levels in safe ranges

You can maintain a healthy equilibrium in your estrogen levels by utilizing some of the following strategies:

- **Make an effort to take control of your weight:** For women between the ages of 55 and 75 who have low estrogen levels, lowering or maintaining their weight may minimize the risk of heart disease. Keeping a healthy weight and maintaining it is associated with a lower risk of developing chronic diseases in general, according to research.

- **Exercise regularly**: If you have low estrogen levels, you could feel like you have less energy to work out. Even

- though estrogen production is lower during menopause and other times in life, maintaining a regular exercise routine is still critical for effective weight management.

- **Eat a well-balanced diet:** It has been demonstrated that diets high in red meat, processed foods, sweets, and refined grains enhance estrogen levels, which in turn may increase the risk of developing a chronic disease. As a result of this, you should probably cut back on how much of these items you consume.

6. Neuropeptide Y

Neuropeptide Y (NPY) is a hormone that is produced by cells in your brain and nervous system. In reaction to periods of fasting or stress, NPY causes an increase in hunger while simultaneously causing a decrease in the amount of energy that is expended.

NPY is linked to obesity and weight gain, which may be because it has the potential to promote food intake.

It is activated in fatty tissue, where it has the potential to enhance fat storage and contribute to abdominal obesity as well as metabolic syndrome, a condition that is associated with an increased risk of developing chronic diseases.

According to research, the same mechanisms that contribute to obesity may also induce an inflammatory response, which further deteriorates existing health issues.

Suggestions for preserving a low level of NPY

Listed below are some pointers that can be used to keep healthy levels of NPY:

- **Exercise:** There is conflicting evidence in the study, but some studies point to the possibility that maintaining a healthy exercise routine can help reduce NPY levels.
- **Consume food that is high in nutrients:** Although further research is required, there is some evidence that diets high in fat and sugar may raise NPY levels. As a result, you might want to think about reducing the amount of sugar and fat-rich foods you eat in your diet.

7. Glucagon-like peptide-1

The production of the hormone known as glucagon-like peptide-1 (GLP-1) in the stomach occurs in response to the consumption of nutrients. It is very important in maintaining steady levels of blood sugar and in preventing feelings of hunger by making you feel full.

The findings of this research point to the possibility that those who are obese have issues with GLP-1 signaling.

As a result, GLP-1 is now being added to drugs, particularly those intended for persons who have diabetes, to lower both overall body weight and the circumference of the waist.

Suggestions for maintaining healthy levels of GLP-1

The following are some suggestions that can assist you in keeping healthy levels of GLP-1:

- **Consume a sufficient amount of protein:** It has been demonstrated that consuming meals high in protein, such as whey protein and yogurt, can raise GLP-1 levels.
- **Think about taking some probiotics**: Even while additional research on humans is required, preliminary evidence suggests that probiotics may raise GLP-1 levels in the body. In addition, before beginning the use of any new supplements, it is highly recommended to consult with a qualified medical practitioner.

8. Cholecystokinin

After eating, the cells in your gut create cholecystokinin (CCK), which is also a hormone that makes you feel full, similar to GLP-1.

It plays a key role in the creation of energy as well as in the synthesis of proteins, digestion, and other biological processes. In addition to this, it encourages the release of the hormone leptin, which makes one feel fuller.

People who are obese may have a diminished sensitivity to the effects of CCK, which may cause them to overeat on a chronic basis. This, in turn,

may result in an even greater reduction in CCK sensitivity, so producing a negative feedback loop.

Suggestions for Elevating Your CCK Levels

The following are some suggestions for keeping CCK levels at a healthy level:

- **Consume a sufficient amount of protein**: There is some evidence that eating a diet heavy in protein may enhance CCK levels and, consequently, a feeling of fullness.
- **Exercise**. Even though research on the topic is scant, there is some evidence to suggest that regular exercise can raise CCK levels.

9. Peptide YY

Peptide YY, often known as PYY, is another hormone produced in the intestines that suppress appetite. People who are obese may have reduced PYY levels, which may cause them to have a stronger hunger, which in turn may lead to them overeating. It is considered that adequate levels play a significant effect in lowering the amount of food consumed and lowering the risk of becoming obese.

Suggestions for enhancing the amounts of PYY

PYY can be maintained at a healthy level in your body by the following strategies:

- **Maintain a healthy and balanced diet:** Consuming a sufficient amount of protein may produce appropriate levels of PYY and a feeling of fullness. In addition, the paleo diet, which includes a generous amount of protein as well as fruits and vegetables, may cause an increase in PYY levels; however, this hypothesis has to be tested further.
- **Exercise:** The study on the relationship between exercise and PYY levels is contradictory, although it is generally accepted that maintaining an active lifestyle is advantageous to one's healt

Chapter 4

The Fats That Cause You to Gain Weight and the

Fats That Cause You to Lose Weight

Dietary fat; It doesn't sound like anything about that is good for you, does it? This is because, in the thoughts of a lot of people, consuming foods high in fat means that you will get well fat.

Several distinct kinds of fat may be found in food, and not all of them are made equal. There is indeed such a thing as "bad" fat, which can play a role in the growth of health problems such as obesity, cardiovascular disease, and high cholesterol.

There is, however, such a thing as "healthy" fat, which is important for your body and can improve your health. A bonus? If consumed in the appropriate amounts, these healthy fats have the potential to assist individuals in better managing their weight.

Because that is a significant amount of information to process, let's divide it up into more manageable chunks.

Which fats should you be eating more of?

The type of dietary fat that you want to have on your plate when you eat is called unsaturated fat. The most familiar sources of this type of fat include foods that come from plants (including vegetables, nuts, and seeds), as well as fatty fish.

Consuming food in moderate amounts that are high in unsaturated fat has been shown to aid in several ways, including the following:

- Reduce the likelihood that you may suffer from heart disease or a stroke.
- Raise levels of healthy cholesterol in your blood while simultaneously reducing levels of bad cholesterol.
- Protect the health of both your brain and your body's cells.
- Increase the body's ability to absorb specific vitamins, such as A, D, E, and K.
- Strive to reduce inflammation.

- Cut down on the chances of dying an early death. (You do realize that this is a huge advantage, don't you?)

Your gut will feel full and content for longer periods when you consume foods high in unsaturated fats, which can help you control your cravings for high-calorie snacks. "These fats are very concentrated sources of calories," the author says. When it comes to stave off hunger, a very small amount can go a very long way.

There are two different types of unsaturated fats, and the primary distinction between them is in their molecular bonding.

The following are the two types:

Monounsaturated fat:

The finest sources of monounsaturated fat are often plant-based foods that have not been refined or processed in any way. The following are some good choices:

- Avocados.
- Nuts like almonds, cashews, pecans, and pistachios are examples of nuts.
- Olives and olive oil go hand in hand.
- Peanuts and peanut butter are also included.
- Seeds such as pumpkin seeds, sesame seeds, and sunflower seeds.

Polyunsaturated fat:

You have almost certainly overheard someone raving about the benefits of omega-3 fatty acids, which are the most prominent figure in the world of polyunsaturated fats. (I'm sorry to disappoint you on the omega-6s, which are another type of polyunsaturated fat.)

Omega-3 fatty acids have been shown to support cardiovascular health, as well as the activity of the brain and vision. In addition to combating inflammation, the high-performing ingredient also helps strengthen your immune system, digestion, and reproduction.

Omega-3 fatty acids are among the most beneficial of all fats, but a significant number of people do not get enough of them.

Fatty fish are among the finest food sources of omega-3 fatty acids. However, there is a possibility that some of these contain high levels of mercury; therefore, I suggest opting for wild-caught salmon,

Bluefin tuna, and herring. (For individuals who do not enjoy eating seafood, foods such as flax seeds, walnuts, and chia seeds are also high in omega-3 content.)

Regarding omega-6s, they have a solid track record that includes doing a good job for overall growth

and development as well as for the health of the brain. The truth is, though, that the majority of us already obtain a very enough amount of omega-6 fatty acids in our regular diet without really making an effort to do so.

Choose to consume more omega-3 fatty acids and less omega-6 fatty acids to better balance your diet and take advantage of the associated health benefits. (By the way, omega-6s are found in high concentrations in canola, soybean, and sunflower oils.)

Which fats should you avoid at all costs?

Which fats should you attempt to stay away from, then? Let's begin with saturated fats, which are likely present in a significant amount of the food you have in your refrigerator. This includes foods that are high in fat, such as fatty cuts of beef and hog, as well as chicken

with the skin. Additionally, foods derived from animals, such as eggs and

complete dairy products (think cheese, ice cream, and butter).

Consuming foods that are high in saturated fat can:

- Put you at a greater risk of developing heart-related conditions.
- Raise your blood cholesterol levels to unhealthy levels.
- Induce inflammation in the body.

According to Taylor, not only are saturated fats hard on your body, but they are also extremely hard on

your weight. "And it's not just that saturated fats are difficult on your body," she says. "These unhealthy fats almost always wind up being a significant source of excess calories, which causes more weight gain over time."

Also, steer clear of trans fats. Artificial trans fat may be significantly worse than saturated fats, which probably explains why the United States Food and

Drug Administration (FDA) prohibited them in 2018. Saturated fats are terrible for you, but artificial trans fat may be much worse. (Before that, it was common practice to include artificial trans fats in the formulation of many processed foods.)

There is a possibility that you might have some outdated products in your cupboard that contain trans fats. In most cases, artificial trans fat can be found hiding in partly hydrogenated vegetable oil, so make sure to check the labels for that.

6 BEST FATS FOR LOSING FAT

Yes, it is necessary to consume fat to reduce body fat. Not the combo of bacon and fries, though. The following items should be placed on your plate.

Have you ever been terrified of eating fat? You have no reason to be worried. The consumption of healthy fats has been linked to a wide variety of health benefits, some of which include a more rapid reduction in body fat. To maintain a healthy metabolism, cell signaling, the integrity of many different body tissues, immunity, hormone production, and the digestion of a wide variety of foods, we require a proper amount of fat (such as vitamins A and D). They make us feel fuller for longer, improve our brain and visual function, and help reduce inflammation throughout the body. They almost always have a wonderful flavor as well.

In addition, we need to keep our overall health in mind while we work to reduce our body fat. The fat loss problem is complicated by

multiple factors, including the function of the brain, the reduction of inflammation, cell signaling, and other metabolic functions.

The following are our top six sources of fat, each of which is loaded with all of the health benefits, as well as the ability to build muscle and burn fat, that you could dream of.

Fish caught in cold waters that were caught wild, as well as fish oils

The fish should have a healthy amount of fat. Omega-3 fatty acids can be found in abundance in oily fish, including salmon, tuna, sardines, mackerel, and trout. Other sources include mackerel and sardines. People should try to consume at least two servings of fatty fish every week, as recommended by the American Heart Association, to help maintain a healthy ratio of omega-6 to omega-3 fats in their bodies. Not to mention all of the other health benefits that come from the DHA and EPA, which are two essential nutrients found in fish that provide a variety of benefits, such as reduced inflammation to recover from your workouts and sore joints, which makes it much easier to continue training the way you need to to support fat loss.

Extra Virgin Coconut Oil

This fat is the most significant nutritional advancement made since butter. Or even bacon (which is not good for you). Coconut oil is an

instant upgrade for numerous reasons; grass-fed butter is wonderful and offers a lot of advantages, but coconut oil has even more advantages. It is extremely versatile and can be utilized in the same ways that butter is, including cooking and spreading. According to a number of studies, consuming coconut oil can help increase your resistance to pathogens like viruses and bacteria that can make you sick and prevent you from engaging in strenuous physical activity. In addition to that, it may also be useful in the fight against candida, fungus, and yeast. If you don't believe that this is beneficial, then you should ask yourself how much fat you have the potential to burn

when you are sick and/or lethargic. Coconut oil has a beneficial effect on our hormones, which helps regulate our thyroid
and blood sugar levels, which are both highly important hormones for fat loss. A physique athlete's best buddy is their hormones. Last but not least, lauric acid is a form of medium chain triglyceride (MCT) that does not get stored as fat and is a fantastic source of energy. This acid can be found in coconut oil, which is a saturated fat.

Extra Virgin Olive Oil

Olive oil has been shown to lower the risk of certain types of cancer, as well as heart disease and blood pressure. Olive oil may reduce the risk of stroke, according to the findings of a recent study that was published in the journal Neurology. The study looked at the effects of using olive oil in cooking and salad dressing. What an excellent

source of nourishment for the mind! Olive oil contains a high concentration of monounsaturated fats, which research has shown can aid in weight loss in people even when no other aspects of their diet or lifestyle
are altered significantly. Imagine then what it has the potential to achieve for people who train hard.

Avocados

When dieting for a competition or trying to get as thin as possible, adding avocados to any recipe that features chicken and broccoli is an excellent way to add taste and diversity without completely derailing your diet. It has a lot of monounsaturated fat, which is good for your heart because it decreases your total cholesterol and assists your body in burning more fat (see No. 3). Additionally, avocados are an excellent alternative to dips that do not offer very much in the way of nutritional value.

Organic Eggs

In your quest to get a leaner body, how many times have you flushed the egg yolk down the toilet instead of using it? Too many, no doubt. This is a mistake of the gravest order because the egg yolk is

loaded with omega-3 fatty acids, B vitamins, choline, and other nutrients that help regulate the brain, nervous system, and cardiovascular system. This is a mistake of the gravest order because the egg yolk is loaded with omega-3 fatty acids.

Even though there are still some who say that eating eggs is unhealthy because of the cholesterol they contain, research has established a correlation

between moderate egg consumption and improved heart health. Not to mention the fact that the cholesterol found in eggs can assist enhance testosterone production, which plays a significant role in both the performance of strength-based exercises and the loss of body fat. In addition, eating whole eggs can assist in increasing feelings of fullness, and studies have shown that eating eggs for breakfast can help prevent the kind of lunchtime binges that can derail efforts to reduce body fat.

Nuts or Nut Butter

Pistachios, almonds, and walnuts are your best bet when it comes to their nutritional value. Pistachios have lutein and zeaxanthin, which are two carotenoids that are essential for eye health. Almonds are an outstanding source of vitamin E, while walnuts are an adequate source of omega-3 fatty acids that are derived from plants. According to research, people who consume nuts daily tend to have a lower body mass index, a lower chance of developing type 2 diabetes, and a lower risk of formulating heart disease. Additionally, nut butter has several health benefits—that is, assuming you can refrain from devouring the entire jar. Just be wary of the added sugars that may be present in certain products. Because it is high in

calories and contains only a trace amount of protein, nut butter is an excellent choice for a munchie while one is on a diet.

***Both quantity and quality are important.**

Chapter 5

Fixing the problem of obesity,

Diet

To lose weight at a healthy and manageable rate of 0.5 to 1 kilogram
per week, the majority of individuals are urged to lower the amount

of energy they consume each day by 600 calories. However, no one guideline is universally applicable.

This means that the average man should consume no more than 1,900 calories per day, and the average woman should consume no more than 1,400 calories per day.

The most effective strategy for achieving this goal is to replace high-energy and unhealthy food options, such as those found at fast food restaurants, processed foods, and sugary drinks (including alcoholic beverages), with healthier alternatives.

A healthy diet ought to include the following:

- an abundance of fresh fruits and veggies

- a plethora of starchy foods, including potatoes, bread, rice, pasta, and others (ideally, you should choose wholegrain varieties)
- milk and other dairy products in some cases
- Some sources of protein other than dairy products, such as meat, fish, eggs, and beans.
- Simply a few bites and sips of foods and beverages that are heavy in sugar and fat.

If you are already overweight, you should make every effort to steer clear of meals that contain high concentrations of salt because eating such foods might cause your blood pressure to rise, which can be dangerous.

To ensure that you do not go over your calorie allotment for the day, you will need to look up the calorie content of every meal and beverage that you put into your body.

Even while it's not required for eateries like restaurants, cafes, and fast food chains to do so, some of these establishments do disclose the number of calories in each serving. When dining out, use caution because the calories in some items, such as burgers, fried chicken, and certain curries and Chinese dishes, can easily add up to more than the daily allotment.

Diet plans and fad diets.

Steer clear of trendy diets that advise you to engage in dangerous behaviors, such as abstaining from food for extended periods or eliminating whole food groups from your diet. These kinds of diets do not work, can make you feel poorly, and cannot be maintained because they do not teach you healthy eating patterns that you can carry with you in the long run.

This is not to imply that any and all commercial diet programs present a health risk. Many are founded on strong medical and scientific concepts and have the potential to be effective for certain individuals.

A responsible diet program should:
- Provide you with information on topics such as the appropriate serving size, making adjustments to one's behaviors, and eating healthy.
- Not be extremely restricted regarding the kinds of foods that you are allowed to consume.
- Be built on attaining progressive and lasting weight loss as opposed to quick weight loss in the near term, which is unlikely to be maintained.
- Diets with a very low-calorie content

Consuming less than 800 calories on a daily basis is the definition of a very low-calorie diet (VLCD).

These diets can result in a rapid loss of weight, but they are not an approach that is appropriate or safe for everyone, and they are not typically suggested as a treatment for the management of obesity.

VLCDs are typically not indicated unless the individual in question has an obesity-related condition that would be helped by significant weight loss in a short amount of time.

In general, very low-calorie diets (VLCDs) shouldn't be followed for more than 12 weeks at a period, and they should only be taken under the guidance of a healthcare professional who is appropriately qualified.

If you are thinking about going on this kind of diet, you should consult with your primary care physician first.

Extra details can be found here.

If you would like additional information regarding diet and weight loss,

Exercise

You can help yourself lose weight by cutting down on the number of calories you consume each day, but staying at a healthy weight requires an activity of some kind to burn off the calories you consume.

In addition to assisting you in keeping a healthy weight, regular physical activity has a wide range of other positive effects on your health. For instance, it can assist in the prevention of and

management of more than twenty illnesses, such as lowering the chance of developing type 2 diabetes by forty percent.

A minimum wage of 150 minutes of workout per week at a moderate level is what is recommendable for adults. This might be broken down into five sessions of 30 minutes each week, as an example. Even exercising for only ten minutes at a time has positive health effects, proving that doing something is always preferable to doing nothing.

Any activity that causes an increase in both your heart rate and your breathing rate is considered to be of a moderate level.

aerobic exercises like fast walking and cycling, recreational activities like swimming and dancing

Alternatively, you may engage in vigorous activity every week for 75 minutes, or you could combine moderate and vigorous activity for 150 minutes.

When you are engaging in intensive activity, it is quite difficult to breathe, your heart beats very quickly, and you may find that you are unable to carry on a conversation. Examples include:

The majority of competitive sports include running as part of their circuit training.

In addition to that, you should perform strength training and balance training twice a week. This could take the shape of going to the gym and lifting weights, carrying shopping bags, or participating in an exercise like tai chi. It is also essential that you get up and move around every so often to break up long periods of sitting (sedentary) time.

Your primary care physician, a weight reduction adviser or the staff at your local sports center may be able to assist you in developing a plan that is tailored to your individual requirements and circumstances and includes targets that are both attainable and inspiring. Begin on a low scale and work your way up slowly.

Discovering hobbies that you take pleasure in and wish to continue doing is another essential step. Motivating yourself to exercise or participate in other physically active pursuits by inviting friends or family members can be a big assistance. Get started right away; it's never too late to get things going.

Learn more about the physical activity requirements for adults as well as the physical activity guidelines for older individuals by doing some further reading.

If you've ever struggled with obesity and want to keep from putting on weight again, you might need to increase the amount of time you spend exercising every day. It is recommended that people engage in physical activity for 45–60 minutes each day at a moderate level. It is achievable that you will need to engage in 60–90 minutes worth of activity on a daily basis in order to prevent the return of your previous obesity.

Your primary care physician or a weight loss counselor will be able to provide you with more advice regarding the kind of activity you should
perform and for how long, taking into account your present degree of physical fitness as well as your specific circumstances.

Additional helpful strategies

There is mounting evidence that demonstrates a greater likelihood of successful weight loss if, in addition to dietary and lifestyle modifications, other weight management treatments are also implemented. This might contain items like the following:

- **Having goals for weight loss that are attainable:** is important because if you are obese, decreasing as little as 3 percent of your total body weight can greatly cut your chance of developing issues associated with obesity.

- **Consuming food more slowly and mindfully:** both in terms of the food itself and the timing of its consumption; for instance, refraining from eating while watching television.

- **Avoiding situations in which you are aware that you may be tempted to overeat;** involving your family and friends in your efforts to lose weight because they can help to motivate you; monitoring your progress by, for example, weighing yourself on a regular basis and keeping a record

- of your weight in a diary; avoiding situations in which you are aware that you may be tempted to overeat; involving your family and friends in your efforts to lose weight;

If you want to modify the way you think about food and eating, getting psychological counseling from a skilled healthcare professional who can help you may also be helpful. Techniques that can be helpful include cognitive behavioral therapy (also known as CBT).

Avoiding weight regain

It is vital that as you lose weight, your body requires less food (calories). As a result, even if you continue to follow a diet after a few months, your rate of weight loss will slow down and eventually level off.

After you have lost weight, if you go back to eating the same amount of calories as before, you will almost certainly gain the weight back. It is possible that if you continue to pay attention to what you eat and increase the amount of time you spend being physically active (up to sixty minutes a day), you will be able to keep the weight off.

Managing the treatment of childhood obesity

Improving a child's diet and using behavior change tactics to encourage increased physical activity are typically required treatment methods for childhood obesity.

Your child's age and height will determine the appropriate number of calories for them to consume on a daily basis. Your primary care physician should be able to provide you with information regarding a suggested daily limit, and they should also be able to refer you to the family healthy lifestyle program that is offered in your community.

Children above the age of five should ideally have at least one hour and sixty minutes per day of exercise with a strong intensity, such as running, playing football or netball, or other similar activities.

Restrictions ought to be placed on sedentary activities like watching television and playing video games on a computer.

If your child develops a complication that is related to obesity, or if it is believed that there is an underlying medical condition that is causing obesity, it is possible that a referral to a specialist who treats pediatric obesity will be recommended.

The use of orlistat in children is not recommended unless there are extenuating conditions present, such as when a child is extremely fat and has a condition that is associated with obesity.

In most cases, bariatric surgery for children is not suggested; however, it might be explored for adolescents with unusual circumstances and who have either reached or are very close to reaching physiological maturity.

Conclusion

Treating obesity is maybe the most difficult task that healthcare providers confront in the modern day. The growth in the prevalence of obesity is associated with increased medical issues. Most adults who develop obesity do so not as a result of a particular medical or metabolic condition but rather as a result of lifestyle behaviors that lead to increased food consumption and decreased energy expenditure. These lifestyle behaviors almost always cause obesity in adults. It is necessary to do further study to understand better why obese people practice certain behaviors and how these behaviors might be modified to attain better long-term weight control.

Efforts should be focused on enhancing personal behavior and environmental variables to avoid obesity or delay disease advancement. Altering and bettering our environment is the most important factor in preventing and reversing this public health disaster, even though the treatment methods for obesity mentioned in this article may be effectively applied to fat persons.